Learning and Enriching
Who I Am

An African American Teen Mother to Be

Denise Corpening

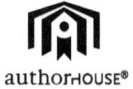

authorHOUSE®

AuthorHouse™
1663 Liberty Drive, Suite 200
Bloomington, IN 47403
www.authorhouse.com
Phone: 1-800-839-8640

First published by AuthorHouse 10/1/2008

ISBN: 978-1-4343-9545-0 (sc)

Printed in the United States of America
Bloomington, Indiana

This book is printed on acid-free paper.

A WEEKLY JOURNAL AND GUIDE TO PREGNANCY AND MOTHERHOOD

Contents

Preface

This weekly journal and pregnancy guide is written for every young African American Mother to Be.

As you think about, write about, and dream about, the beautiful life growing inside of your womb, you begin to realize that you have so much more life to live, things to experience and opportunities to learn. Hope and prayer gives vision to what life may have in store for you. Knowledge and determination helps you obtain those visions. You *can* reach out and touch your successes and defeat your challenges by beating the odds and becoming whatever you set out to be in life. Don't ever give up. Believe in your strengths.

I reach back in my thoughts and bring to mind my personal experiences as a teenage mother. I remember the tears strolling down my cheeks, during my pregnancy as I finally had to accept that I was going to be a mother. What would I do? How can I handle it all, school, pregnancy, and parenting? At times it wasn't easy. But I never gave up my dreams and motivation to make a difference in my life and the life of my newborn. Looking at and holding my baby son for the first time helped confirm the reasons I needed to advance my life and be the best that I could be.

I did it. So can you.

This journal is dedicated to every mother's struggles and every mother's dreams.

Share your thoughts and dreams with your loved ones and others who care. It will make a difference to help you prepare and achieve your goals.

Denise

Acknowledgment

I wish to acknowledge my three sons, Mark, James and Armaad. Their births taught me how to love unconditionally and gave me more gratitude and joy than I could have ever imagined. Their being gave me the power and motivation to reach for my highest capabilities. Much love and appreciation to my wonderful husband, Ron, for *always* being my source of support. His patience and understanding is invaluable. Last but not least, I want to thank my dad, John, my friends, Lisa, Donnie, Karen, Jackie, Pat and all of you (you know who you are) for believing in me. You are my girls! Thanks.

-- *Denise Corpening*

Introduction

This week to week guide through your pregnancy and birth is a great source of information for you but is also meant to provide a window in and capture your feelings and realities of pregnancy.

Learning and Enriching Who I Am will provide you with a blend of the physical and emotional changes of pregnancy sprinkled with some of the everyday African American culture, views and beliefs that many of us live by daily. This book is "topped" with a peek into the uterine walls that your baby now lives in for a look at the weekly growth and development of your baby. By the conclusion of this journal you will feel closer to confronting your personal feelings and experiences and more prepared to face the ultimate challenge – Motherhood. Month_____ Year_____

Week One - Four: *Wow...I'm pregnant!*

Feeling as if you are carrying the entire load of the world within is common. You are not alone. It happens to thousands of young expectant mothers. Many young African American women experience fear, anger and denial when learning of their pregnancy for the first time. Often times the pregnancy was unplanned and undesired. All of these feelings may feel overwhelming but can be very normal. Always remember, there *is* help available when you need it. Seek out available resources. You don't have to do it alone.

How was the pregnancy confirmed? _____

_____

How did you feel when you found out? _____

_____

Did you tell anyone? If not, why? _____

_____

_____

Notes_____

_____

_____

_____

_____

_____

_____

_____

Month_____ Year_____

Week 5: *While you were sleeping…..*

Often times a good night sleep can make things look brighter. Despite how gloomy things may appear at first, sleep can be a beginning to looking at things with a fresh outlook. Depending on your own individual circumstances, how you personally handle situations and what support systems are available to you, maybe a good night's sleep may be a start to help relieve or lessen your stress. Aim for eight hours of sleep per night.

Are you able to sleep? If so, do you find you are able to think about the pregnancy and how to deal with it? Are your thoughts becoming brighter now? _____

_____

_____

_____

_____

_____

Are you faced with so much stress that you are finding it difficult to move forward? What are your plans?

_____

_____

_____

_____

Notes _____

_____

_____

_____

_____

_____

_____

_____

_____

_____

_____

_____

_____

_____

Month_____ Year_____

Week 6: *Has the pregnancy become "real" to you yet?*

Do you believe that if you face things head on, the power of strength will take over? Strength often comes in numbers. For many decades African American families and communities have taken pride in coming together during troubled times. Don't be too ashamed to reach out for help when you need it.

Do you have someone to lean on? Who is that someone?

_____

_____

_____

_____

_____

Are you able to confide in and talk to that person? What are some of the things that you have discussed with that person?

_____

_____

_____

_____

_____

_____

_____

_____

_____

_____

_____

_____

_____

_____

Notes _____

_____

_____

_____

_____

_____

_____

Month_____ Year_____

Week 7: *Let's take this journey together*

Has someone in your family had a recent dream of fish? That is an old wives tale in the African American community that means someone in the family is pregnant. These tales are often passed on lovingly through the *matriarch of the family for years to come. Someone in your family may already suspect that you are pregnant. Go to them and talk about your feelings and plans.

Now that you have your support person by your side, you can plan the journey for your pregnancy. If your pregnancy has not been confirmed **or** has been confirmed by a home pregnancy test, it is now important to see a doctor. Have you scheduled a doctor's appointment for your first* prenatal visit? If not, call your doctor's office or clinic today.

_____
_____
_____
_____
_____

Don't have a doctor? You can call your local hospital or ask family and friends to help you find one.

*A prenatal visit is a visit to a doctor who specializes in the care of the expectant mother. Early and regular prenatal care is important for the health and growth of you and your baby.

Notes

_____
_____
_____
_____
_____
_____
_____
_____
_____
_____
_____
_____
_____
_____
_____
_____
_____
_____

Month_____ Year_____

Week 8: *While you are waiting......*

Seeing the doctor for the first time could take a couple weeks, depending on the office or clinic's schedule. There are many things that you can do before seeing the doctor, to keep you and your baby healthy. A well balanced diet, exercise, avoiding stress and plenty of rest and sleep are just a few. Never take any over the counter medications or other medications without talking to your doctor or nurse first. Say no to alcohol or drugs.

Did you know that the first couple months of pregnancy, your baby's organs are being formed and are completely formed by 8 weeks? This includes the heart which is now beating.

_____
_____
_____

Avoiding certain infections and diseases are important in the first few months. Remember, to report all infections to your doctor. Your doctor will test you for any existing infections present that you may not be aware of, at your office or clinic visit.

Notes

_____
_____
_____
_____
_____
_____
_____
_____
_____
_____
_____
_____
_____
_____
_____

Month_____ Year_____

Week 9: *Changes are taking place.......*

This week, many things are taking place within your body. In your uterus the *umbilical cord is formed with two large blood vessels that carry blood to and from the *fetus. You may be noticing some physical and emotional changes in your body. *Fatigue, nausea and vomiting, heartburn, soreness of your breasts are very common discomforts in early pregnancy.

Did you know that you should always report any problems or symptoms to your doctor or nurse, even if you think they are normal?

_____

_____

_____

Some types of foods or different food smells can play a role in causing more discomforts of pregnancy. Avoid foods that do not agree with you. Have you noticed any changes in the foods that you like to eat or any special cravings?

Notes

_____

_____

_____

_____

_____

_____

_____

_____

_____

_____

_____

_____

_____

_____

_____

_____

_____

_____

_____

_____

Month_____ Year_____

Week 10: *But I like fast food and my mamma's home cooking!*

Good nutrition is very important in pregnancy. That does not mean you have to give up everything that is good to you! But, to make sure your baby is getting the proper *nutrients to grow, you may have to make some changes or add to your usual meal plan. Drinking 8-10 glasses of water a day and eating fruits and vegetables is a great start. Many African American families use a large amount of butter, fats (cheese), and sugar in their cooking, which has proven unhealthy and can cause large amounts of weight gain in pregnancy.

Did you know there are a number of low fat and low sugar food products available that taste pretty good? Have you tried any? Which ones?

_____

_____

_____

What is your starting pregnancy weight? Have you talked with your doctor about weight gain (or loss) and how much you should gain during pregnancy?

Notes

_____
_____
_____
_____
_____
_____
_____
_____
_____
_____
_____
_____
_____
_____
_____
_____
_____
_____

Month_____ Year_____

Week 11: *Generations of Food*

You haven't had a meal until you sit down to a meal at an African American home. We have had traditions of good home cooking with lots of family centered at the table. This can be a time to get involved with the family menu. This can also be a time to just "talk" to family. After dinner is also a good time to take a short walk with family members.

Have you ever heard of the word "*Pica*?" It means "an unusual non food craving". Eating laundry starch, dirt, and clay are all forms of pica. They do not serve any nutritional value. Do you have any of these cravings? Try to substitute with other healthier choices. What are some of your favorite food choices?_____

_____

_____

Did you know that you should **never "diet" in pregnancy**? Many African American teen mothers want to keep their same body figures and want to avoid "looking pregnant" and gaining weight. This is one reason that selecting good diet choices are important. Healthy diet choices provide good nutrients to you and your baby and have fewer calories to help control weight gain. Your doctor may order Prenatal vitamins, Iron supplements, Folic Acid and calcium to help balance your diet during pregnancy. _____

_____

_____

Your doctor or nurse will weigh you at every office visit. Write your monthly and weekly weights in your journal.

Notes _____

_____

_____

_____

_____

_____

_____

_____

_____

_____

_____

_____

_____

_____

Month_____ Year_____

Week 12: *I'm trying to take it all in, but it's hard!*

There is so much going on. Woo. Your body is changing and you have some good and some bad days, mood changes and heavy emotions. You are still trying to come to terms with the pregnancy. Some days you don't feel like you can handle everything, pregnancy, school, family are all becoming hard to deal with. It's OK. We all feel like this from time to time. Take a deep breath, turn on your favorite song, eat a special meal or call someone you can talk to. African Americans, especially women are often known for their power to overcome. A favorite saying, "This too, will pass" means over time you can adjust.

Think of things that come to mind that make you feel good. What makes you feel good?
_____
_____

Can you picture yourself as a new mother in your mind? If yes, what do you think will make you a special mother?
_____
_____

You are entering your second *trimester of pregnancy. Your baby is developing its own sex organs, but it is still too early to tell rather it is a boy or girl. There are so many developments taking place inside of you. It is truly a miracle!
It is always a good idea to gather information and read pregnancy related books and materials that can help you understand the growth and development of your baby.

Notes
_____
_____
_____
_____
_____
_____
_____
_____
_____
_____
_____
_____
_____

Month_____ Year_____

Week 13: *Time is ticking on*

Things are settling down. You are beginning to take hold and pay close attention to the pregnancy and the changes in your body. You may start to notice the size of your *abdomen getting larger as your fetus is growing in your *uterus. Stretch marks may start to form on the abdomen, thighs and behind as the uterus grows. African American traditions may include applying different lotions (cocoa butter, Shea butter) to the skin to prevent or lighten stretch marks. Stretch marks are caused by a break or tear in the connective layer of the skin.

Linea Nigra is the medical term for the brown line that appears down the middle of your abdomen. Mother to be of all races may notice this skin change but for African Americans the line tends to be darker and more visible. Can you see the beginning form of Linea Nigra?

_____

_____

Breast changes are common in pregnancy. Developing a larger size and darkening of color around the nipple can occur. Make sure you are wearing the proper bra size as your breasts enlarge.

Notes

_____
_____
_____
_____
_____
_____
_____
_____
_____
_____
_____
_____
_____
_____
_____
_____
_____

Month_____ Year_____

Week 14: *I've had my doctor visit.*
I am even more confused.

Your first prenatal visit can be filled with lots of questions and testing. This will help the doctor and medical staff to give you and your baby the best care. Health questionnaires are important to identify any existing problems or diseases that may complicate this pregnancy. It is important that you are truthful when asked about any health problems, diseases or mental/social issues that you are experiencing.

Did you know that diseases/health issues and social habits of the family and father of the baby may be just as important in the growth and development of your baby? Are you aware of any health/social issues of the father of the baby? If so, did you inform the doctor?_____

_____

_____

_____

Did you know at (14) fourteen weeks your baby may have learned to suck his or her thumb and your baby may be the weight of a letter (1.52 ounces)? These images can be noticed on a *3d Ultrasound. Have you had an ultrasound yet? When?_____

_____

_____

_____

Make sure you are asking questions of your doctor and nurses to help understand your pregnancy. Sometimes, you may feel that even after something is explained, you still do not understand fully. There are a number of outside resources and information available to assist you and clarify unanswered questions.

Notes

_____

_____

_____

_____

_____

_____

_____

_____

_____

_____

_____

_____

Month_____ Year_____

Week 15: *Tests, tests and more tests*

Urine samples, blood pressure/pulse/temperature, blood tests, *physical assessment exam which includes a *vaginal/cervical exam, measuring the size of your abdomen and checking the fetal heart rate and movement are some of the "routine" tests that are done at the early prenatal visit.

Did you know that there are some testing that can identify problems/diseases specific to different races and cultures, example Sickle Cell trait and disease? Does anyone in your family carry the Sickle Cell trait or disease? _____

_____

_____

Have you ever heard the African American *old wives tale that a fast baby heartbeat is a Girl and a slow baby heartbeat is a Boy? Have you heard your baby's heartbeat yet? What do you think, boy or girl? _____

_____

Are you feeling some little flutters in your tummy yet? Your baby is kicking and twisting around in there and you may be feeling that. But if not, <u>don't panic, you will feel it soon!</u> Pay close attention and write down when you feel those flutters!

Notes

_____
_____
_____
_____
_____
_____
_____
_____
_____
_____
_____
_____
_____
_____
_____
_____
_____
_____

Month_____ Year_____

Week 16: *Ultrasounds and other procedures done in pregnancy*

Many doctors will perform a bedside ultrasound during your early pregnancy, usually between 16 to 20 weeks. This ultrasound is done to find out information on the growth and development of your baby. Ultrasounds also give the doctor an image of the uterus, placenta and other pelvic organs. Sometimes, your doctor will order a more "specialized" ultrasound that can give them additional information on fetal organs.

Many African American mothers to be believe that ultrasounds should be done routinely at every office visit. This may be a way to reassure that the fetus is doing well and may possibly give them a "**sneak peek**" of the sex of the unborn.

The decision *to do or not to do* an ultrasound is based on any information that the doctor is looking to gain from performing the procedure. Every pregnancy is different. It is "OK" if your doctor only does one, two, three ultrasounds, or doesn't do any at all. It is entirely up to you and your doctor. Ultrasounds should not be considered "routine".

Have you had an ultrasound? When? _____

_____

Alphafeto Protein (also known as the "Triple Screen") is a simple blood test that is drawn from you to check for levels of a protein found in the fetal liver and released into your blood. This test screens for certain abnormalities such as *Spina Bifida and *Anencephaly. This test is done between the 15th and 18th week of pregnancy. Results are usually available in (1) week. Please ask your doctor to explain what high or low levels of this test means.

Have you had yours done? What were the results?

Notes

_____
_____
_____
_____
_____
_____
_____
_____
_____
_____
_____
_____

Month_____ Year_____

Week 17: *Being "Real", can help you!*

Just as I have mentioned the importance of making your first prenatal appointment, <u>it is just as important to keep all regular scheduled prenatal appointments with your doctor.</u> Many of you may have difficulty arranging transportation for your visits. There are some local organizations that may provide assistance or arrange a *referral to get you to your appointment.

If you are having difficulty making your prenatal visits due to transportation issues have you informed your doctor? If yes, were you offered any referrals or help?

_____

_____

Many of us have difficulty or are embarrassed to tell our doctor or nurse other things that go on in our lives that we may feel are "personal". Belief of many people in the African American culture often tend to hold things inside, believing that things will straighten out on its own or others "will not understand". However, social issues that directly affect you can also cause stress. *Stressors are known to effect the pregnancy, i.e. domestic/sexual abuse, *incarceration (jail) of a family member/significant other, lack of money. Talk to your doctor openly. Don't be afraid or embarrassed. He or she can lend an *objective opinion. Many times, your doctor and nurse can give you very useful information that can help your situation. Use your support person or call M.O.M, LLC when you need *reinforcement to discuss a difficult subject. Do you have any social problem(s) that you are having a hard time talking about? If yes, what can we do to help? **Call US.**

_____

_____

_____

Guess what? Your baby weighs about 4.97 ounces and is about 5.12 inches long. WOW!

Notes

_____

_____

_____

_____

_____

_____

_____

_____

_____

Month_____ Year_____

Week 18: *The list goes on and on*.........

By now, your doctor has probably discussed or given you a list of <u>Do's and Don'ts in pregnancy</u>. When looking over the list, many things you can probably live with, but there are a few that will take some getting used to. Let's talk about a couple of things that may be "*hard to do*" for the African American teen or young mother to be.

1) **Perm or hair color/treatments** – Most of us appreciate a good looking hairdo! Many doctors or nurses will ask you to prevent from using any hair treatments that involve chemicals for the 1st *trimester. Wear your baseball hat; if you need to, for the first 3 months, then, you can rock your new style!!!

2) **Drink 8-10 glasses of water a day** – if water is not your favorite thing use lemon or other flavors to boost the taste. Try to stay away from sugar and high calorie sweeteners. A favorite of the African American culture, Kool-Aid, is OK as long as it is not overly sweetened. Water is the best choice by helping provide fluid *hydration to your placenta and baby.

3) **Avoid alcohol, cigarettes and drugs** – If you are using any street or recreational substances, please inform your doctor. They can have a very serious effect on you and your baby. Now is a good time to get involved in a program to help you stop. If you are having a problem with alcohol, cigarettes or illegal drugs, there are many organizations that can help. **What substance(s), if any, are you using**? _____

_____

_____

Have you reached out for help in the past? If so, what happened?

Notes

_____
_____
_____
_____
_____
_____
_____
_____
_____

Month_____ Year_____

Week 19: *He is your "Baby Daddy", but is he <u>there for you</u>?*

While it is important, if possible, to have a "support person" by your side, it does not necessarily have to be the "Baby Daddy". Many African American teens and young woman remain in unhealthy and abusive relationships (mental, physical or sexual) because he is the "father of the baby". These relationships can become complex and even dangerous and can cause harm to you, the pregnancy and the baby. Don't feel "pressured" by him or your peers to remain in this type of relationship. This may require involvement by your parent(s) or other professionals that can help sort things through. Other support persons have your best interests in mind and are willing to help. If you and the father of the baby have a "positive and working" relationship, by all means if you both agree, he should be included in your prenatal course and progress of your pregnancy.

Is your relationship with the "father of the baby" (FOB) a good relationship? Do you communicate with him about the pregnancy? If so, does he attend prenatal visits with you?

_____
_____
_____

If problems exist in your relationship with the FOB, have you told anyone? Who? Have they become involved? What happened?

Notes

_____
_____
_____
_____
_____
_____
_____
_____
_____
_____
_____
_____

Month_____ Year_____

Week 20: *Are we there yet? Half way!*

20 weeks is not only half way but also a point of many physical milestones during your pregnancy. If you have unclear of what you have been feeling, you are now pretty sure of the movement you are feeling inside. *Quickening = the first time fetal movement is felt. Many other physical changes are also taking place. If you are carrying a girl, her eggs are beginning to develop. Brain nerve cells and intestinal development of the fetus is also occurring. This may be a time that the doctor or nurse may notice (elevations) or increases in *your* blood pressure. BP elevation related to the pregnancy, also called Pregnancy Induced Hypertension is a complication found in many pregnancies of young African American women.

Do you know your most recent BP? Remember to ask your doctor at each scheduled prenatal visit and write your BP in your journal.

_____

_____

There may be other symptoms that are associated with Pregnancy Induced Hypertension such as headache, blurred vision, swelling and *epigastric (chest) pain. If you are feeling any of these, let your doctor know immediately.
Have you experienced any of these symptoms? Which one(s)? Did you report the symptoms to your doctor?

Notes

_____
_____
_____
_____
_____
_____
_____
_____
_____
_____
_____
_____
_____

Month_____ Year_____

Week 21: *How big is my baby now?*

Your doctor will start to measure your uterus at every prenatal visit. This simple measurement, done with a tape measurement, gives your doctor information on the growth of your uterus. This measurement is called a *fundal height. If there is a time that your doctor notices that your uterus is not growing adequately in relationship to the weeks of your pregnancy, he or she may decide to perform an ultrasound to look closer at the growth and development of your fetus. The term, Intrauterine Growth Restriction (IUGR) is used when the fetus is known to be smaller or the growth has been restricted or slowed. One known fact is that poor diet and nutrition of mom, which leads to lack of weight gain, therefore may increase the risk of inadequate nutrients (vitamins and minerals) reaching your fetus.

Have you spoken with your doctor and discussed all the important nutrients needed in pregnancy to help keep you and your baby healthy? _____

_____

_____

Did you know, depending *on your age*, you may need extra protein, iron, calcium and folic acid supplements to support you and your fetus's growth and development?

There are many resources available that can help you understand good nutrition in pregnancy and making better dietary choices. If you doctor finds problems in your diet or the growth of your baby that need more attention, he or she may ask you to see a * Dietician. A Dietician can give you more detailed information on diet and nutrition.

Have you made any food choices lately that were really *good* for you lately? What choices did you make? That is great. You deserve to be **congratulated!** Eating well is often hard to do when there is so much fast food around.

Notes

_____
_____
_____
_____
_____
_____
_____
_____
_____

Month_____ Year_____

Week 22: *I'm feeling it now, boy, do I feel pregnant!*

Your baby weighs close to a pound now. Now is a great time to begin talking, reading and singing to your baby. He or she can hear you! Often times in the African American culture, families begin to get excited and are really looking forward to new addition to the family. As your abdomen is growing and you are now starting to "show", you may notice even complete strangers may want to rub your tummy. *Effleurage is a form of circular touching and rubbing of your abdomen that causes relaxation. Avoid wearing tight clothes that prevent you from moving freely and restricting your abdomen. Many expectant moms no longer wear "maternity clothing" but now wear normal everyday clothing during their pregnancy.

By this point in your pregnancy your doctor may have already given you the results of your lab tests taken early on in your pregnancy. The type of lab (blood) tests ordered may vary based on your doctors' orders. Some "routine" blood tests ordered in pregnancy are *Rubella, *RPR, *HIV, and *Blood group and type. *Chlamydia and Gonorrhea culture swabs are also done in early pregnancy.

Has your doctor performed these blood tests? If so, were you informed of the results? Were they normal?

_____

_____

_____

Were any additional tests performed?

Notes

_____

_____

_____

_____

_____

_____

_____

_____

_____

_____

_____

Month_____ Year_____

Week 23: *I never thought about that…*

We have discussed not taking "over the counter medications" without asking your doctor first. Another type of these medications may include "remedies and herbals". To some in the African American community, remedies and herbals are largely used. There may be longstanding cultural beliefs that certain remedies are safe and helpful for pregnancy aches and discomforts. Beliefs such as taking castor oil and Magnesium Citrate for constipation or BC powder for headaches are among the few medication choices that many African American families have lived by for generations. If your family has specific cultural remedies that are used, write them down and tell your doctor on your next prenatal visit. Your doctor will inform you if this "remedy" or medication is safe to take in pregnancy.

Have you heard a similar saying by someone in your family? "*Me and my mother took it, and it didn't hurt us*". Many times this may be a true statement but certain medications may have different effects and complications to some.

Do you know of any "family remedies" that are used in your family? What are they?

Notes

_____
_____
_____
_____
_____
_____
_____
_____
_____
_____
_____
_____
_____
_____
_____
_____
_____
_____
_____

Month_____ Year_____

Week 24: *I am always feeling bad. Is this normal?*

Most expectant moms experience "common discomforts in pregnancy". Pregnancy is unique to every mother, so the gestational stage in which she experiences discomforts and the severity of the symptoms may also differ. Common discomforts include nausea & vomiting, fatigue, heartburn, *gingivitis, headache, backache, muscle cramps, varicose veins, and urinary frequency to mention a few. Even though these discomforts may be considered *normal* in many instances, you should still report this to your doctor. You doctor will better determine if your symptoms and experience is normal *for you and your baby.*

Did you know that headaches are often considered normal in pregnancy *but* a headache that continues on with little or no relief is **not normal and should be reported to your doctor immediately?** Have you had a headache that just does not go away? If yes, did you report it to your doctor?

_____

_____

Urinary frequency (frequent urination) can be caused by the baby's' position putting pressure on your bladder but can also be a symptom that should be reported to your doctor. Have your experienced urinary frequency and noticed that you are emptying your bladder in small amounts when you go? Did you report this to your doctor?

_____

This is a milestone week for your baby. This is the official week that your baby is considered *viable. Your baby now weighs about 1.3 pounds and is 11.8 inches long.

Notes

_____
_____
_____
_____
_____
_____
_____
_____
_____
_____
_____
_____

Month_____ Year_____

Week 25: *Some things are just private.*
I don't want to talk about them.

Some "private" discomforts in pregnancy are understandably hard to discuss with your doctor. Vaginal discharge is one of the discomforts that happen to most young women once puberty is reached. In pregnancy, there may be an increase in this vaginal discharge caused by changes in the *hormone levels. Frequent bathing and wearing a panty liner may help control the problem. Never use a tampon or insert anything into your vagina. This can cause a vaginal infection. Infections (vaginal or urinary) may cause complications in pregnancy. Any change in the amount or color of a vaginal discharge or itching should be reported to your doctor to *evaluate for infection. Many African American woman have practiced "*douching" and believe this is the best way to get rid of the discharge. Douching can cause other complications and should not be done without an order from the doctor.

Have you noticed a change in your vaginal discharge? If so, have you informed your doctor?

_____

_____

_____

Early evaluation and treatment of infection is the best way to prevent further complications in pregnancy.

Guess what? Your baby can now make a fist and would grab things put into his or her hand. Wow!

Notes

_____

_____

_____

_____

_____

_____

_____

_____

_____

_____

_____

_____

Month_____ Year_____

Week 26: *How could this happen?*

Some infections can be diagnosed as Sexually Transmitted Diseases (STD). Chlamydia, Trichomonias, Herpes, Condyloma (Warts) and Syphilis are all considered STD's. Symptoms of these infections can go unnoticed or be very mild. Many times the first symptoms that are noticed with a STD are changes that start in the vaginal area. It may be an abnormal bump or growth found, some itching or an odor noted. These symptoms or any changes in your body should be openly discussed with your doctor. The best way to prevent contacting a STD is to avoid unhealthy sexual behaviors (multiple sexual partners and unsafe sex). Always practice safe sex! Sexually Transmitted Diseases are known to cause further complications in pregnancy and should be treated immediately.

Did you know there currently is no cure for Herpes? Once diagnosed with Herpes you will have periodic flare ups of uncomfortable *lesions. There are medications available that may ease the discomfort and prevent frequent flare ups. If you have a flare up of lesions on your vagina at the time of childbirth, your doctor will choose to deliver your baby by *Cesarean Section (C/S). This will prevent the baby from passing through the birth canal and developing the disease.

Have you noticed any unusual bumps or growths to your vaginal area? If so, please report the symptoms to your doctor.

_____

_____

Your baby eyes are opening and beginning to blink. Your baby weighs about two pounds now.

Notes

_____
_____
_____
_____
_____
_____
_____
_____
_____
_____

Month_____ Year_____

Week 27: *But, I don't have Diabetes....*

Between 24 and 28 weeks of pregnancy your doctor will screen you for *Gestational Diabetes (high blood sugar). A (1) hour Glucose Challenge test is a sugar solution that is given to you to drink over 5 minutes. This tastes like a sweet soda pop. One hour later your doctor or nurse will draw blood from your arm to check your blood sugar level. Your doctor will want to see how well your body processes sugar. This test will give a reading (value) and you will get the results of the reading in a few days. If the value comes back abnormal or too high, your doctor will ask you to come back for a (3) hour Glucose Tolerance test to see if you really have gestational diabetes. Often times, you will pass the 3 hour test and not have gestational diabetes. Many older African Americans refer to Diabetes as "Sugar" or "Sugar Diabetes".

Being diagnosed with Gestational Diabetes does not mean you will continue to be a diabetic throughout life. Gestational Diabetes is a health problem of pregnancy and usually goes away after childbirth. Once diagnosed your doctor will discuss the best treatment plan for you such as diet, exercise or *insulin therapy. If diet control is recommended, you will probably meet with a Dietician to discuss the best meal plans for you and your baby. Good nutrition is important to your baby too!

Have you had your 1 hour glucose screening or 3 hour glucose testing? If so, what were the results?

_____

_____

Babies born to diabetic moms are usually larger in weight. These babies may have complications from their mothers' diabetes. Talk to your doctor about the complications of Gestational Diabetes.

Notes

_____

_____

_____

_____

_____

_____

_____

_____

_____

Month_____ Year_____

Week 28: *What is Preterm Labor?*

Since most expectant moms have had some discomforts during the pregnancy it is often difficult to determine when aches and discomforts become important and should be evaluated by your doctor. Preterm labor can begin as early as 20 weeks through 37 weeks of pregnancy. Preterm labor that is not treated or controlled can lead to delivering prematurely, before the baby is fully developed. Preterm labor can have a number of symptoms, some very noticeable, others that you may not be aware of. African Americans have a higher rate of babies born premature. One way to help control premature births is to recognize the symptoms of preterm labor and get early treatment. Severe back ache, lower abdominal pain or regular contractions (tightening or balling up of the uterus), thigh pain, vaginal bleeding or change in your vaginal discharge can all be symptoms of preterm labor and should be reported to your doctor. Symptoms left untreated could cause changes or opening of your *cervix that can lead to premature delivery.

Did you know that babies born prematurely may spend days or weeks in the *Neonatal Intensive Care unit (NICU) receiving care for lung, brain and heart problems? These babies can also have complications and birth defects that last a lifetime.

Have you noticed any symptoms of Preterm Labor? If so, what are the symptoms? Did you report the symptoms to your doctor?

_____
_____
_____

New moms desire having a healthy baby that can come home from the hospital *with them*. Babies that are carried to full term, (37-40 week gestation) have the *best chances for a healthy start at life*.

Notes_____
_____
_____
_____
_____
_____
_____
_____
_____
_____

Month_____ Year_____

Week 29: *What happens if my water breaks?*

Your baby is surrounded by a bag of water also called *Amniotic Fluid*. This fluid protects the baby from injury and also helps to keep a normal fluid temperature around the baby. When the bag of water breaks the baby no longer has this needed protection. We normally expect "Rupture of Membranes" (bag of water to break) to take place when the pregnancy is full term or at the start of labor. Often, the bag of water does not break on its' own and is broken artificially by the doctor when the mom is in labor. Infection is an important concern of your doctor when your water breaks prematurely (20-37 weeks of pregnancy). Both you and your baby can develop an infection. Based on individual factors involved with your pregnancy, your doctor will decide on the plan of care for you and your baby and discuss the options for delivery. If you suspect that your water has broken, you should check for the color, amount and odor, if any and report to your doctor immediately. Amniotic fluid is usually clear-whitish looking and may have little white speckles within.

Did you know many moms have reported that their water has broken and it is actually urine? It is not uncommon to have pressure on your bladder from the baby and growing uterus which may lead to "wetting your pants". Don't be embarrassed. Labor and Delivery nurses see this all the time.

Have you felt any fluid or suspect that your bag of water has broken? If so, did you call your doctor immediately?

_____
_____

Did you know that your water bag is truly like a "water balloon? You can have just a small "leak" of amniotic fluid in your water bag and it can sometimes seal itself over.

Notes

_____
_____
_____
_____
_____
_____
_____

Month_____ Year_____

Week 30: *Is bleeding a true emergency?*

Any bleeding in pregnancy should be considered an emergency and you should seek medical attention right away. That does not mean bleeding always has a *bad outcome*. Bleeding happens in pregnancy for many reasons. Spotting in pregnancy can be common for some moms but unusual for others. Some report spotting after a recent cervical exam or recent sexual relations. Similar to amniotic fluid, bleeding should be reported to the doctor by taking notice of the amount of bleeding, the color ((pink, bright or dark red), if clots are passed, or if any pain is present with the bleeding. Certain complications with the *placenta can also lead to bleeding episodes throughout the pregnancy. Many times it is the episode of spotting or bleeding that will alert your doctor that there may be a problem and this will prompt your doctor to look at the placenta on ultrasound for further evaluation.

Did you know that the use of cocaine in pregnancy is *one* of the causes of a severe disorder that causes the placenta to "tear apart" and cause severe pain and bleeding? This is known as ***Placenta Abruption.**

Notes

_____
_____
_____
_____
_____
_____
_____
_____
_____
_____
_____

Month_____ Year_____

Week 31: *Boy, my feet are swelling!*

It is not uncommon to notice *some* swelling in your legs, feet and hands. Many times this swelling may be a result of the long periods of standing or excessive heat related to the weather. You may often notice more swelling of your legs, feet, ankles and hands during the summer months. However, there is some swelling that is of concern. This swelling will leave an "indentation" or a dent in the area of swelling once you press on and release your fingers. This means that fluid is being *retained or pooled in that area. Swelling, also known as *edema,* can also be one symptom of a disease in pregnancy called *Preeclampsia. Preeclampsia is diagnosed when there is a combination of high blood pressures, swelling, and *urine protein. Headaches, blurred vision and *epigastric pain are other symptoms associated with this disease. Most importantly, this disease can be very serious and can cause complications for both you and your baby. If you experience any of these symptoms, report them to your doctor. Your doctor will want to watch you closely and order other tests to determine the best plan of care for you.

Have you had any signs or symptoms of Preeclampsia? If so, what symptoms have you experienced?

_____

_____

_____

Did you know the most preferred position for lying in bed is the *left side position?* This increases blood flow through your major blood vessels to the heart and uterus. Also, a quiet, dim lighted room works best to help calm you and control your blood pressure.

Notes

_____

_____

_____

_____

_____

_____

_____

_____

Month_____ Year_____

Week 32: *How much longer? I'm ready.*

As the time nears, it is common to have the feeling to "get this over with" and have your baby. You are feeling more uncomfortable as you abdomen is growing and growing and growing! You may feel more restless and it is becoming harder to sleep at night. Your family and friends may begin to comment and tease you about the size of your abdomen or make remarks about other things that are noticed about your pregnancy. Older African American *matriarchs often have known someone in the past who has delivered a baby prematurely. It is common to hear them say "My family or friend had a baby at 7 or 8 months and that child is doing fine". As we are aware, some babies *may do well* if delivered early, but there are also babies that don't do as well and have lifelong effects and problems. That is why we want your baby to stay in your uterus as long as needed (full term) to receive the benefits that will increase the chances of a healthy baby. But don't be disappointed, your childbirth is getting near!

Are you getting excited as the time is getting closer? Have you started thinking of needs for the baby, clothes, car seat, stroller, etc?

_____

_____

_____

Your baby has assumed the "fetal position" with his or her legs bent into the chest as it is getting more cramped inside. The baby lungs are fully formed and baby is "practice breathing". If your baby is a boy, testicles have formed and may begin to move into the scrotum and if it is a girl, she has already developed her own "eggs". Isn't that amazing!

Notes

_____

_____

_____

_____

_____

_____

_____

_____

_____

Month_____ Year_____

Week 33: *I have so much to do!*

It is a good idea to stay busy with other activities throughout your pregnancy. School, work and activities with family and friends can really help to pass the time and before you know it you are planning and thinking about other things you have to do before the baby comes. Preparing for the birth of the baby involves planning and detail. First time moms often depend on family and friends for knowledge, support and ideas. Planning for the baby also includes preparing for the labor and delivery and the actual day the birth will take place. For the first time you may begin to think of what type of delivery you will have, a vaginal delivery or Cesarean Section Delivery, what type of pain control you may want or even how many people you may want to be with you during your labor and delivery process. All of these are important issues and require much thought and planning.

Have you and your doctor discussed the type of delivery that you are expecting to have? If so, do you have knowledge and understanding about the delivery procedure?

_____

_____

_____

_____

Do you have a list prepared for items that you will be taking to the hospital? Have you packed your bag yet? Do you have your doctor and emergency numbers available for you and your family? It is a good idea to start now.

Notes

_____

_____

_____

_____

_____

_____

_____

_____

_____

_____

Month_____ Year_____

Week 34: *I'm still waiting…..*

Even when busy planning for the birth of your baby you can't help but feel tired, often, feeling fat and ready for that special day to come. You want your "shape" back and your body to yourself. You may have even heard an old wives tale that suggests having a baby in the eight month of pregnancy *gives the baby a better chance* of *survival* than carrying the baby through the ninth month. This is untrue but if the baby *is born* during this month, there is usually a good chance of survival. While your baby is developing its final growth touches before arrival, you too, can be fine tuning final plans. One good option is to educate and prepare for the actual childbirth experience by registering for "Childbirth classes". You can usually pick up information pamphlets at your doctor's office or at your local hospital. These classes are helpful in understanding what to expect during labor and delivery and help explain available options to the mother in labor. Many young African Americans expectant mothers may not be aware of these classes or how to register for them and may miss the opportunity to expand their childbirth knowledge. Ask your doctor or nurse at your next office visit.

Have you registered for childbirth preparation classes? If yes, plan to attend every scheduled class. Jot down the scheduled location and dates of classes. What have you learned in class, pain control, epidurals, breathing and relaxation, pushing, newborn care?

Notes

_____
_____
_____
_____
_____
_____
_____
_____
_____
_____

Month_____ Year_____

Week 35: *Believe it or not; I am getting it together!*

All kinds of things are running through your mind now. Who will I use as a *Pediatrician, will I breastfeed or bottle feed, do I want an *epidural, will I have the baby circumcised if it is a boy, do I need to *pre-register at the hospital, who will I use for child care, are just a few of many questions that may still be undecided. It takes time and help to make these decisions. Depend on the advice of your doctor, nurses, family and friends. Other "sisters" who are already moms are great *resources. If you are attending childbirth classes there may be other moms or couples that you may ask as well. When you are making decisions on selecting a Pediatrician or Childcare providers, make an appointment(s) to go out to see or "interview" the person before your decide. Your baby's health and safety is a priority to you. Making sure that you are leaving your baby in safe and responsible hands is very important. Your baby is depending on you!

Write down some appointments or scheduled visits that you have arranged.

_____
_____
_____
_____
_____

Your baby is getting lots of antibodies from your immune system to help prevent him or her from developing certain infections and diseases. This is a temporary immunity *but* breastfeeding your baby after birth can help extend this immunity.

Notes

_____
_____
_____
_____
_____
_____
_____
_____
_____

Month_____ Year_____

Week 36: *36 weeks and counting....*

By now you are visiting your doctor or clinic more often and usually the last month of pregnancy you will have weekly appointments. As the time gets closer to birth your doctor will likely perform additional tests and exams to evaluate you for the *impending delivery. Your doctor or nurse will examine your *cervix. Normal changes may start to take place in your body as Mother Nature prepares for the labor and birth of your baby. Labor begins when your cervix starts making normal changes, dilatation (opens), effaces (thins) and the baby starts moving down in the birth canal. You may have a vaginal swab performed for *Group Beta Strep. This is a routine culture that is done on most expectant mothers. Your doctor should inform you of the results of the test, positive or negative. Your doctor may also order other tests at this point of your pregnancy that will help determine how the baby is doing inside the uterus and how well the baby will do during labor. These tests are called * BPP or Biophysical Profile and *NST or Non Stress Test.

Has your doctor performed a "cervical check" at your visit yet? Did your doctor report rather your cervix was dilated or effaced? If yes, what was the value?

Notes

_____
_____
_____
_____
_____
_____
_____
_____
_____
_____
_____
_____
_____
_____
_____

Month_____ Year_____

Week 37: *The time is here!*
I thought it would never come.

Have you started feeling that "surge of energy"? Do you have this extreme urge to clean out closets, under beds and areas of the house that you normally wouldn't clean? What about, noticing some tightening and releasing of your abdomen or the baby "balling up" more frequently? Have you noticed some "pinkish mucous" (normal show) on the toilet tissue when you wipe? All of these can be early signs and symptoms that your body is *preparing* for labor. These symptoms are important and should be reported to your doctor *but do not* necessarily mean that you will have your baby in the next couple hours or days. These symptoms can occur as early as weeks before actual labor begins. Keep in mind, every woman is different and no two women will have the same symptoms, complaints or experiences. African Americans mothers, friends, grandmothers, church members and others, may readily share their personal experiences with you and may offer many suggestions at this time. These suggestions can range from everything from when to call the doctor, when to go into the hospital, what's normal or not normal, to ways to handle your birth experience. Although most supporters mean well and are sharing information to the best of their knowledge, following their advice should be combined with your own personal knowledge and awareness. This is <u>your</u> experience.

At this gestational period, your baby has now taken the "birth position", with his head down, facing your back. The average weight may range from 6 to 9 pounds and measure from 17 to 22 inches.

Notes

_____
_____
_____
_____
_____
_____

Month_____ Year_____

Week 38: *Okay, it's time. I'm ready.*

It's finally here. Are you experiencing regular contractions in your uterus? Have you timed the contractions and know how close together they are coming? Contractions should develop in a pattern over time and get stronger and longer lasting over time. Has your water broken? If so, did you notice the time your water broke, the color of the water or if the water had an odor. These are all things your doctor will want to know to make an initial assessment and decide whether you should go into the hospital now or wait until later. You know your body best, so stay in tune to the changes taken place. If you are experiencing pain and are unable to keep account of the contraction pattern, ask your support person or others available to assist you with timing. It is also important to inform the doctor if you experience vaginal bleeding and how much. As we discussed earlier, a normal mucous show may be considered normal but excessive bleeding, like a menstrual period, may be abnormal. Wearing a panty liner or pad to the hospital can make it easier when explaining just how much bleeding is occurring. Often times, when reporting vaginal bleeding and your bag of water breaking, your doctor will request to see you at the hospital immediately for evaluation.

Write down the type of symptoms, times and other notes related to your labor experience.

Notes

_____

_____

_____

_____

_____

_____

_____

_____

_____

_____

_____

_____

Month_____ Year_____

Week 39: *I'm at the hospital. Now what?*

So many things take place once you arrive at the hospital. While many of the things that take place are routine, other things that may occur are specific to the individual mother to be, her prenatal course and her doctors' plan of care. Routinely, you are taken to your room and placed on a monitor. An "External Fetal Monitor" electronically monitors the baby's heartbeat and the uterine contractions that you are having. Usually, an "IV" is started to help provide hydration to you and baby while in labor. Most doctors do not let you eat solid food and allow you ice or liquids when you are in labor. It is a good idea to eat a small "light" meal before going to the hospital. That should not include your momma's fried chicken, spaghetti or other "heavy" foods. These types of food tend to increase your chance of "throwing up". Your doctor or nurse will check your cervix. Your cervix can be "closed" (not dilated or open) or could range from 1cm (finger) to 10cm (fingers). You and your nurse should be discussing pain control options during your early admission. Your doctor will write an order on your chart as to when it is "OK" to receive medication or your epidural. Sometimes your doctor may want to hold off on giving you an epidural until your labor is "active". This is something you should discuss with your doctor prior to going into labor. Once your cervix dilates to 10cm, you can now begin pushing. Your nurse should instruct you on "how to push". Pushing usually takes time and commonly can take up to 2-3 hours for a first time mother. This is the time to have your support person at your bedside helping you push.

How was your labor and pushing experience? Were you prepared? Did it meet your expectations?

Notes

_____
_____
_____
_____
_____

Month_____ Year_____

Week 40: *But I have been pushing…*
Why do I need a C/S?

Sometimes, despite good efforts of pushing, the baby does not come down in the birth canal enough for delivery. Your doctor may request a C/S delivery (Cesarean Section) performed. This involves an incision (cut) into the uterus to remove the baby. There are a number of other reasons that your doctor will perform a C/S. Before a C/S is decided upon, your doctor will discuss the reason and possible complications of the procedure with you and your support person. You should always receive a "reason" for the procedure. In most hospitals you are required to sign a "consent" form stating that you fully understand the reason and complications of the procedure. A C/S is a surgery or operation and usually requires that you will remain in the hospital an extra day or so, more that giving birth vaginally. A C/S may also cause more discomforts and commonly will take you a little longer to move about freely. However, it is very important to get out of bed when permission is granted and move about. This helps to decrease the chances of developing some complications that could happen after surgery.

Whether a C/S or a vaginal delivery; the goal that all moms aim towards is the birth of a healthy baby. A baby, which in their eyes is the most beautiful and perfect human being alive. A baby to give love; and receive love back.

Congratulations! *You are an African American Mom. This is just the beginning to a long life of love and joy!*

Name: _____

Date of Birth: _____

Time: _____

Hospital: _____

Doctor: _____

Sex: _____ **Weight:** _____ **Length:** _____

Conclusion

Having a baby can be the most loving and rewarding accomplishment of a mother's life but is commonly faced with many feelings of rejection, fear, denial and anger. Far too many times, the young African American pregnant teen feels she has nowhere to turn and no one who can hear her cries for help. There can be so many unresolved issues at hand ranging from health and wellness, culture and lifestyle, family and relationships, and education onward through the everyday challenges of motherhood and growth.

While we use the term "conclusion" for ending the chapters of this guide and possibly other chapters in our lives, we must conclude that adolescent, teenage and young adult pregnancies will continue to occur in every walk of life. We *can* and *will* continue to promote pregnancy awareness and prevention to every teenager regardless of racial, social or economic background. What *can* and *will* make a difference is the way in which we offer non judgmental support, resources and guidance consistently to our expectant mothers.

Often family members, social organizations, churches, schools and other leaders in the community may want to help and may even try to help but have fallen short in ways of offering help. Our young African American pregnant and parenting teens must be lead by example, using advancing education and informational approaches that can be readily received.

It's never too late. Let's hear the cries for help. Show we care and build trust. Our African American moms and babies need us!

It's not about them. It's about us all!

"Talk to Me"

A personal guide to understanding and using words to communicate

Abdomen – stomach, hold the uterus
Alpha Fetoprotein testing – screening test used to determine neural tube defects of the fetus
Amniotic fluid – bag of water surrounding fetus
Anencephaly- an abnormal development of the forebrain of the fetus
Blood group and type- mother's blood type and group – example: **A (group)** positive (type)
BPP (Biophysical Profile) – a test used to determine fetal well being, combination test
Cervix- opening to the uterus
Chlamydia – a sexual transmitted disease
Circumcision – removal of the foreskin of the baby boy penis
Diagnose – to determine a condition
Douching – inserting a fluid into the vagina, used to promote cleanliness
Edema - swelling
Effleurage – a circular movement of hands, rubbing, touching of the abdomen
Epigastric – upper area of abdomen/chest that causes gastric discomfort – symptom associated with Preeclampsia
Evaluation – to look over, review
Fatigue – a state of feeling tired
Fetal heart rate (FHR) or Fetal Heart Tones (FHT) – a fetus heartbeat
Fetus – a development stage of the unborn – after 8weeks gestation embryo matures – called fetus
Fundal height – measurement of top of uterus to pelvis – determines growth of uterus
Gestation – age of unborn - weeks or months of pregnancy
Gestational Diabetes – a problem stabilizing glucose that is first recognized during pregnancy.
Gonorrhea – a sexually transmitted disease
Group Beta Strep (GBS) – an organism found in the female genital track that may cause severe infections in the neonate
GTT (Glucose Tolerance Test) - 1 hour test used for Gestational Diabetes
Hormone levels – levels within the body that responsible for changes that take place during pregnancy
Hydration – to provide fluid
Hyperglycemia – high levels of blood glucose (sugar)
Impending – awaiting, in the future
Incarceration – locked up, in prison
Insulin Therapy – used to control elevated levels of glucose in diabetes
Matriarch – female leader in families
Neonate – name used for infants from birth to 28 days old
Neonatal Intensive Care Unit (NICU) – higher level nursery that provides care to neonates
Non Stress Test (NST) – a test done to determine well being of fetus
Normal Show – bloody drainage, may be mucous, that may be sign of beginning labor
Nutrients – proper intake, vitamins, minerals needed for nourishment
Objective opinion – opinion that is not biased, straight forward
Old Wives Tale – A tale that may not hold complete or any truth
Pediatrician – a doctor who takes care of infants and children
Physical Assessment –to evaluate the physical being and make a calling
Placenta – "afterbirth" in uterus, attached to the umbilical cord, provides nourishment to the fetus
Placenta Abruption – a disorder of the placenta that may cause bleeding and pain – associated with taking cocaine
Preeclampsia – disease in pregnancy that has symptoms of high blood pressure, swelling and protein in the urine, usually diagnosed after 20 weeks gestation
Prenatal – course before birth of baby

Pre-register – to sign up for admission to hospital before actually being admitted

Preterm Labor symptoms – symptoms of, develop of impending labor between 20 – 37 weeks gestation

Preterm Labor – actual labor that starts between 20 – 37 weeks gestation

Quickening – aware of, feeling movement of the fetus for the first time, often between 18-20 weeks gestation

Referrals – recommendations, for care

Reinforcement – to give back up, support, and strengthen

Resources – a source of information

RPR – a test for Syphilis, test done in early pregnancy

Rubella – German measles, an infectious disease. Test done in early pregnancy. May cause severe effects in the fetus

Spina Bifida – a fetal defect of the spine – vertebrae fails to close – testing done by Alphafeto Protein in early pregnancy

Stressors – concerns, feelings, things that cause or increase stress

Syphilis – a sexually transmitted disease

Trimester –3 month period of pregnancy – 3 trimesters of pregnancy

Urine protein – urine tested for presence of protein in Preeclampsia

Viable – a certain gestational age that fetus is considered able to survive outside of uterus

About the Author

Denise is a Registered Nurse and currently resides in the Columbia, SC area with her husband. She has spent the last 28 years as an Obstetrical nurse and women's educator. Experiencing motherhood as an African American teen, her passion continues to advance efforts in providing education and support to other young African American pregnant and parenting teens.

www.ingramcontent.com/pod-product-compliance
Lightning Source LLC
Chambersburg PA
CBHW052014280526
45793CB00005B/977